OVERALL HEALTH

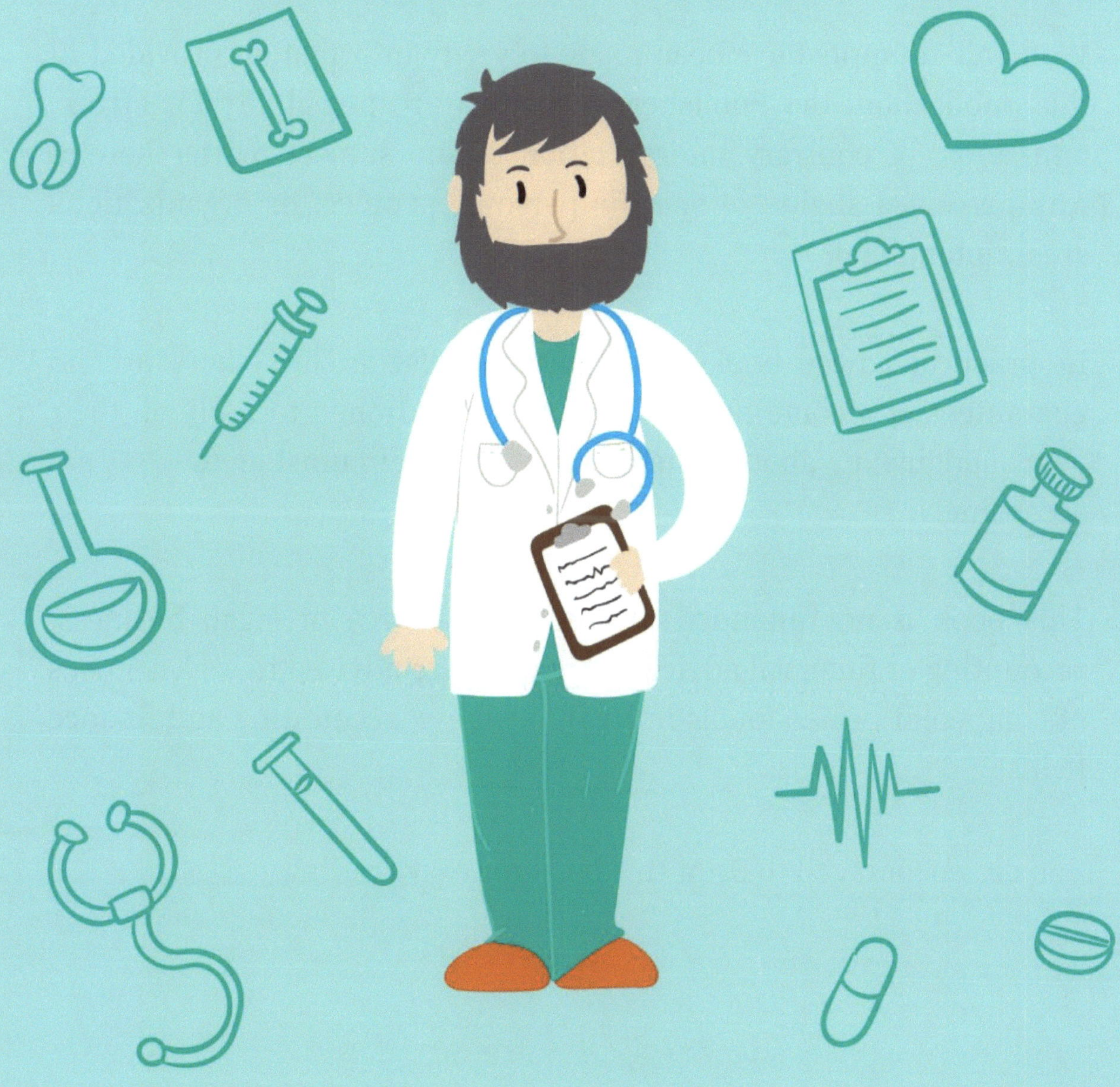

Terms and Conditions

LEGAL NOTICE

The Publisher has strived to be as accurate and complete as possible in the creation of this report, notwithstanding the fact that he does not warrant or represent at any time that the contents within are accurate due to the rapidly changing nature of the Internet.

While all attempts have been made to verify information provided in this publication, the Publisher assumes no responsibility for errors, omissions, or contrary interpretation of the subject matter herein. Any perceived slights of specific persons, peoples, or organizations are unintentional.

In practical advice books, like anything else in life, there are no guarantees of income made. Readers are cautioned to reply on their own judgment about their individual circumstances to act accordingly.

This book is not intended for use as a source of legal, business, accounting or financial advice. All readers are advised to seek services of competent professionals in legal, business, accounting and finance fields.

You are encouraged to print this book for easy reading.

Table Of Contents

Foreword

Engaging ourselves in physical activities is very important regardless of our age and status in life. This is because staying healthy doesn't need a requirement to be able to start. Exercising daily will help us improve our overall health and reduce the risk of any illness. There are few notable benefits if you engage in physical exercise. To name a few, here's the list.

1. It can increase the strength of both bones and muscles

2. It can reduce body mass, keeping it lean and healthy while eliminating body fat.

3. It improves mental health.

4. It can significantly reduce the feeling of anxiety, stress and depression.

5. It supports holistic approach to achieving overall health.

Overall Health

Chapter 1:

Synopsis

Further added benefits can be gained if you engage in a more vigorous type of exercise routine. Studies show that people who exercise daily for longer periods of time, utilizing additional dynamic physical exercises, will likely have more health benefits compared to those who exercise less.

The Basics

For kids, it is best that they begin benefitting from physical exercise at a very young age so that as they develop to adolescent and adulthood they will sustain the value of physical exercise. Additionally, it is very important that they engage in physical activities as it can maintain a healthy body weight. Kids that don't exercise and don't have any other physical activities will likely become overweight. Also, too much of sedentary activities such as playing video games, watching TV programs, surfing the net and the like will increase the chance of becoming obese. Therefore, it is recommended to introduce physical exercise to kids as early as possible for them to stay away from unhealthy activities.

As a final note to achieving healthier bodies, it is critical that we chose the physical activity that best suits us. We need to understand that we have different body types and health conditions, and for that reason we need to know which physical activity can give us the utmost benefit. Talking to the experts will help us identify the right kind of exercises that we can perform daily.

On the other hand, in our effort to lose weight we sometimes skip our meals to speed up the weight losing process. However, by doing this we are sacrificing our health. We don't need to do that. We just need to understand that losing weight is just a matter of burning enough calories that we consumed through our activities. Thus, starting a good physical exercise can well take care of that.

Chapter 2:

The Basics On Physical Health

Synopsis

The act of reading this article demonstrates that you are ready to be physically healthy. However, the greatest challenge of staying fit is not the vigorous exercises or the preparation of a well-balanced food. It is the commitment that you have for yourself that makes all these things about staying fit become extremely difficult.

Create Good Physical Health

Most of us have the intention of staying healthy, but not all of us can sustain healthy living. This is the reason why a lot of self-help tools were made including this article as it can help you continue and eventually achieve your health goals.

To be able to carry on with this seemingly difficult task, it has to be perceived as something you do with no questions. We do these things because we believe that it is important and that we cannot live a day without doing it. The same concept applies when we decide to exercise every day. We need to have that mindset that exercising is the missing piece that will complete the process of staying physically fit and without it our other efforts will not suffice.

Learning the basics of physical health will help you understand what is it that you want to achieve and how it will benefit you. To begin with, there are four basic components of physical health.

1.   Cardiovascular endurance - This can be taken care of with activities like swimming and running. Enhancing this component will improve the oxygen and nutrients supply in the body tissues and at the same time remove stored waste in the body.

2.   Muscular strength - This can be improved with various weight lifting and stretching activities. Enhancing this component will help

you to have stronger muscles that can respond quickly with less effort.

3.   Muscular endurance - This can be enhanced through daily pushups as it can effectively strengthen the arms and shoulder muscles. Enhancing this component will improve the ability of the muscles to withstand repetitive contractions.

4.   Flexibility - This can be improved with regular stretching as it can enhance the tractability of your muscles. Enhancing this component will improve your body's capability of moving your joints as well as using your muscles in their full range.

Having these fundamentals in mind, it is best that your exercise program must include activities that can take care of the four components in order for you to achieve optimum results. As a general guide, make sure that you start your workout with a good warm up and end it with a calming cool down. Also, try not to overwork your body, avoid doing hard exercises consecutively for the whole week.

Chapter 3:
The Basics On Eating Right

Synopsis

Eating right means feeding your body with the right amount and types of food needed to survive each day. When you eat nutritional food you are letting your body absorb the energy that it needs to provide you with more stable energy and moods throughout the day.

Healthy Foods Healthy Life

As you live your daily life, you can plan out a diet that is healthy but also tasty. You don't need to starve yourself to be idealistically thin.

You just need to eat right and exercise regularly to achieve a well-balanced healthy mind and body. The key is moderation.

In all cases, whether or not it is about health or career, strong decisions always play an important role. Once you decide and commit yourself to staying healthy and eating right you are bound to achieve it. The first step to do that is to have a successful mindset about what you are planning.

If you will believe that that you can achieve and maintain a well-balanced diet, it will happen. Just do it in small and gradual steps so that you will not feel that you are obligated to do it. When you are happy with what you are doing, things become easier and eventually it become part of your system.

The goal of healthy eating is for you to maintain a healthy diet that you can sustain for a lifetime. Therefore, after knowing which foods are best for your health, set a standard and food moderation. Remember, the goal is long term and not just achieving your ideal weight. Thus, make sure to set moderation in good balance of fat, carbohydrates, fiber, protein, vitamins and minerals for you to achieve a well-balanced and healthy body.

On the other hand, when you eat, take time to grind your food. It will not only let you savor the food, it will also improve digestion. Also, when you think that you have already consumed enough, stop eating! Normally it takes a few moments for your stomach to get a signal from your brain that you are already full.

Eating fruits and veggies in every meal will complete your healthy diet as they are rich in antioxidants, fiber, vitamins and minerals while giving you low calories in the body. In general, fruits and vegetables that are deeply colored have more concentrated vitamins and minerals that can give you more benefits. Consuming five slices is enough for a day.

Also, get enough healthy carbs and avoid unhealthy fats. Whole grains are the best source of healthy carbs that can give you lasting energy for the entire day. It is also rich in antioxidants and phytochemicals that can help you stay away from cancer, coronary heart disease and diabetes. On the other hand, eating healthy fats will help you nourish your cells, brain, heart, hair, nails and skin. Additionally, it can help you sustain a good mood and reduce the risk of cardiovascular diseases and also helps you avoid dementia.

Chapter 4:

The Basics On Exercise

Synopsis

Most of us know how important exercise is in our daily lives is. It is one of the backbones of our overall health. To add, physical exercise is proven effective in reducing stress as well as emotional setbacks. When you exercise on a regular basis you are more likely to stay healthier, happier and composed most of the time compared to those who rarely exercise.

Keep Fit

Despite the fact that we know how important exercise is, still we cannot find time to do it and stick to our exercise schedule on a regular basis. Why do we need to exercise anyway? What do we get out of it? Read on to understand more about the concept and benefits of exercise. Regular exercise has countless benefits, below are the most noted.

1. An effective way to lose weight while maintaining a healthy and lean body even as you age

2. Effective in maintaining bone mass

3. Lowers bad cholesterol, blood sugar and blood pressure

4. Effective in reducing stress and enhancing sleep

5. Maintains good cardiovascular health, energy, flexibility and a good physical image.

The above mentioned are the most known benefits of exercise. Many people are under the impression that when they are doing their regular activities such as gardening, sweeping, washing the car, cleaning the dishes and the like, they are already exercising and expect to get the same benefits of structured exercise. This is not the case!

Unfortunately, your daily activities are different from structured exercise, where you can expect great results. Your daily activities will just help you burn some calories and stay active. Thus, if you want optimum results, you should do both on a regular basis.

To get a good start, see your doctor and ask for advice as you might have some limitations when you exercise. In most cases however, exercises are safe to perform. Limitations only apply to people who are suffering from chronic diseases, heart problems, arthritis, bone problems, high blood pressure, respiratory problems and the like.

Once you have done the initial steps, find out which exercise best suits you and make it a routine. Do not strain yourself. Do it gradually but regularly. Make sure that you enjoy what you are doing, because if you don't you will eventually lose interest in doing it. You may try changing your routine and try other fitness exercises as long as you can benefit from it. This should be done to reduce boredom in the long run.

Chapter 5:
The Basics On Mental Disorders

Synopsis

A mental disorder is defined as a condition that affects how a person feels, thinks and behave with or without the influence of other people around them. The person who is suffering from a mental disorder might show some mild to severe signs of mental disability, depending on the person's condition. Most of the sufferers finds it hard to cope with even the simplest routines and demands from work and home.

Develop A Healthy Mind

There is no exact cause of mental illness. However, studies show that mental malady is triggered by one of the following factors or combined psychological, biological, hereditary and environmental problem and not really a personal weakness. Thus, in most cases this condition cannot be alleviated by simple self-discipline as it apparently needs the intervention of doctors and medicine.

Following the cause is the types of mental disease. Mental conditions can be treated effectively using the right approach. Thus, knowing its type can help enhance the recovery process. Below are the most known types of mental disorders.

Psychotic disorders – It is described as having a distorted thinking and awareness pattern. Its most common symptom is hallucinations. The person with a psychotic disorder may experience weird images and sounds that they perceive as true events despite their clear notion of delusion. One known example of a psychotic disorder is schizophrenia.

Personality disorders – These disorders are characterized by extremely stubborn personalities that causes the person or the people around to feel stressed and upset. This is the reason why people with personality disorders always encounter problems at work, school, home and even personal and social relationships with people. This is because the way they think and behave is extremely different from the normal individuals. Some examples of this condition are obsessive-compulsive personality disorder, paranoid personality disorder and antisocial personality disorder.

Mood disorders – These disorders are also known as affective disorders. They are described as having a relentless feeling of sadness or happiness or fluctuation of the two extreme emotions. For instance is the condition of being extremely happy to feeling extremely sad. Examples of this disorder are bipolar disorder and depression.

Anxiety disorders – A person with an anxiety disorder responds to certain situations with great fear and horror resulting in serious nervousness, sweating and rapid heartbeat. Examples includes but are not limited to specific phobia, panic disorders, generalized anxiety disorders and social anxiety disorder.

Addiction disorders – These are characterized by uncontrollable urges to perform things that are detrimental to our own self and others. Examples are stealing, gambling, alcohol and drug dependency.

Eating disorders – These disorders are characterized by extreme attitudes, emotions and behaviors relating to food and weight. Examples of this include Bulimia Nervosa, binge eating disorders and Anorexia Nervosa.

Chapter 6:
The Basics On Stress

Synopsis

Stress is defined as a reaction to something that bothers us physically, mentally and emotionally, which as a result affects our equilibrium. Therefore, stress is innate and can be triggered when something adverse happens. When a stressful event takes place the fight/flight response is triggered causing the adrenaline and cortisol in the body to rise to keep us alert and alive.

Relax!

Having a small amount of stress is good but keeping it for a long period of time can significantly affect our overall health. While stress is unavoidable, the best way to prevent it to linger more is to change your reaction towards stress. How will you do that?

You need to understand stress and why it has to be present in our lives. Stress has several types and levels. Therefore, it makes sense that we get affected by it in so many different ways. For us to manage it effectively we must understand first what types of stress we are experiencing. That way we can condition our mind and body to expel stress as quickly as possible.

Stress should not be perceived as something bad at all times because in life stress can either be good or bad. What makes stress becomes bad is when we allow it to stay in us for a long duration. The good side of stress when present in moderation is the energy that it gives us that keeps us alive and stimulated to do our tasks. Recognizing the good stresses from the bad ones will allow you to use it to your advantage.

Our health can be greatly affected by stress when taken for granted. It can cause us to get sick every so often. Not only that, "chronic stress" can also affect our mental health which could possibly lead to emotional instability. Before that happens, you have to stop the madness before it ruins you completely.

Research also shows that stress has an effect on your physique. This is because when you have stress overload, chances are you will care less about yourself. You won't pay much attention to your looks and worse you will not care about your eating pattern and the type of foods that you are consuming which can cause change to how your body processes the food. If this happens, your weight and body figure will be greatly affected.

Stress can also affect our way of life and relationships. When we are stressed we are likely to feel that there is never enough time for us to complete our responsibilities. As a result, involvement becomes less and you hardly see your friends and family. Also, since stress can make someone moody, you might hurt your loved ones because of your erratic mood.

Chapter 7:
The Basics On Mental Health

Synopsis

Generally, one needs to have a healthy mind to be able to do things right. Our mental power helps us become effective in what we do. Further, it plays an important role in our lives to help keep things in order. Mental health is a general term. However, it relates to the overall condition of our mind where our level of psychological health is high and at the same time free of any mental disorders.

Happy Mind, Happy Life

A person's ability of staying happy and enjoying life can also be measured by their mental health. The reason for this is that our mental capacity can greatly affect our emotions, thus our expressions and reactions are also affected.

When your mental health is poor your judgment on things is also poor because your mind cannot function rationally. Being mentally ill will change the way you look at life and react on it. Most of the time you are emotionally unstable, which is why a lot of people who are not having a healthy state of mind becomes an easy target of depression and other forms of mental disorders.

Our mental health can be affected by a lot of things including our physical make up, environment, work, relationships and genetics. Today, a lot of studies have been made purposely to give high priority and importance on how a person achieves mental wellness for the reason that people nowadays need to cope with the world that requires healthy people, both physically and mentally to be able to live a bountiful and creative life.

In general, the areas of our life that can be deeply affected by our mental condition are our spirituality, work, relationships, emotions, relaxation and self-direction. Moreover, we have to understand that even if we are mentally and emotionally healthy, it does not always mean that we will never experience hassles from the uncontrollable and unforeseen issues. However, a healthy mind and spirit will help us cope with any challenges with a better outlook which can help us to stay focused, flexible and result driven.

To be able to maintain good mental health, we need to prevent any risk factors that can trigger mental and emotional instability. Also, when facing a difficult situation, stay focused and identify the root cause of the problem so that you will know how exactly to deal with it.

Finally, since all of us want to have a beautiful and peaceful life, let us all allow ourselves to relax and fill our lives with positive people and always choose to have constructive relationships rather than the opposite.

Chapter 8:
The Basics On Spiritual Health

Synopsis

Our spirit is technically not part of our physical attributes, but it is considered a significant part of our wholeness as human beings. Our body works in harmony with our mind and spirit, thus each of them can affect one or the other. Having said that, if you are concerned with your physical and mental health you also need to be equally concerned with your spiritual wellbeing.

Get In Touch

Many of us are not aware that having a healthy spirit allows our body to heal faster as it can contribute good energy while you are in the process of healing. While it is not considered the actual cure, it is still considered a part of your treatment since it can greatly help you manage any pain and complications that usually go with an illness.

Spiritual health can be attained when you're life is in perfect harmony. Meaning, you find comfort even when you are in pain and you find hope even when you are in despair. Life is completely different when your spirit is healthy.

Sometimes when we are seriously ill, we tend to forget our beliefs and just let it die because we feel that our sickness is eating us up. But what we do not know is that when we are spiritually healthy, we have more strength to combat sicknesses of any form simply because we are complete beings. Therefore when our body, mind as well as our spirit is in harmony, our chance to recover fast is high.

On the other hand, if you feel that your spiritual health is not in good shape, take time to reflect and look at how you live your life in a wider perspective. Stop for a while and listen to your inner soul and feel its calmness. That way you can well understand the very essence of your life, what is it that makes you feel complete and where exactly it is that you find your inner strength. Above all, keep a positive outlook on life and you will see how your life will change for the better.

Chapter 10:
The Benefits Of Maintaining Overall Health

Synopsis

Maintaining overall health will give you several long term benefits. For kids, performing regular exercise will help them develop strong bones, healthy joints and muscles. While for adults, consistent workout will help them eliminate excess fat to give way to a leaner body. Furthermore, it decreases the risk of having diabetes, fractured bones, heart problems, specifically colon cancer and other types of severe sicknesses. Research shows that physical exercise can also help reduce stress and depression by about 50%, plus the fact that it gives immediate results.

The Good Stuff

Another way to sustain overall health is to combine regular exercise with dietary supplements. This is because nowadays, it is very difficult for each of us to really eat a balanced diet, considering the high demands of both personal and professional jobs.

Dietary supplements can fill the needed nutrients that our body needs even in times that we are unable to meet the desired balanced food intake. What's good about it is that people have become more aware of the benefits of wellness products including food supplements. Therefore, you can easily choose dietary supplements that will best fit your needs.

Most of the food supplements that are made available in the market today include herbs, vitamins, minerals and amino acids. Such elements are considered as the most needed substances of our body as it provides a lot of physical benefits.

In addition to the general benefits of food supplements are other accompanying benefits that a specific supplement can provide, such as supplements that can enhance the mood of an individual to be able to cope with different levels of stress.

For pregnant women, taking folic acid can significantly reduce the chance of having a child suffering from spina bifida. Niacin produces good cholesterol as well as omega-3 which reduce the levels of triglycerides.

In ancient times, people discovered some plants and herbs that helped them stay physically and mentally healthy. This is why scientists of the modern times researched more and developed herbs and supplements as they wanted the modern people to experience the benefits that the ancient people are benefiting from, even if people nowadays no longer eat naturally nutritious food.

Wrapping Up

Ultimately, for you to be able to take care of your overall health, you need to stick to your routine that enriches your physical health and combine your effort with the necessary supplements that you need for you to achieve a well-balanced diet, body, and mind. This way you are confident because you are taking the essential steps to improve your overall well-being. You will feel great about yourself as you see the transformations go under way. Enjoy life at a much happier pace and learn to relax. Use the steps you have just learned to get yourself in the best mental and physical state so that you may live a peaceful life. Good luck!